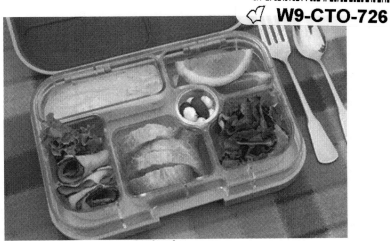

Photo courtesy of www.yumboxlunch.com

Yum!

Healthy Bento Box

Lunches for Kids

Sherrie Le Masurier

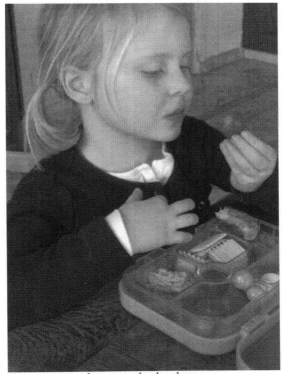

Photo courtesy of www.yumboxlunch.com

Healthy Eating for Kids

Preschool to Age 10

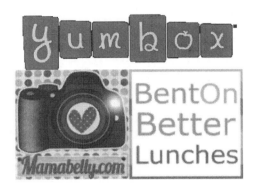

Photographs courtesy of

www.yumboxlunch.com
www.mamabelly.com
www.bentonbetterlunches.com

ISBN-13: 978-1482741667

ISBN-10: 1482741660

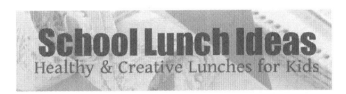

Table of Contents

Introduction

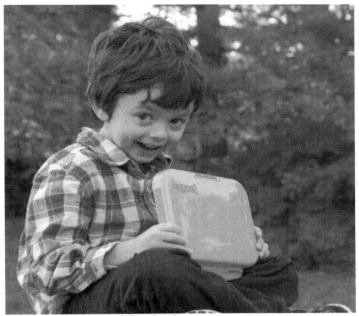

Photo courtesy of www.yumboxlunch.com

Welcome to **Yum! Healthy Bento Box Lunches for Kids**, where you'll discover some creative tips and ideas for packing bento box styled lunch boxes.

This quick and easy digest book discusses nutritional foods for preschoolers and primary grade children.

Inside you'll discover how eating out of a bento box is like opening a treasure chest. It's all in what you pack in it and how you present it. From notes to fun little treats, eating out of a bento box can be a real adventure.

The truth is healthy eating is simple and straightforward once you have the right tools and ingredients. You'll no longer have any excuses for packing boring lunches, as this book also offers up some good menu item ideas even for the pickiest of eaters and for those days when you're getting low on groceries.

Among the best things about bento box styled lunch containers is that the food doesn't touch and it can be served up the way young children typically like it best – finger style.

While some kids prefer all their menu items cut up into bite-size pieces, others simply like the variety a bento box offers.

Healthy and creative bento box lunches also don't have to be time consuming to prepare. We'll share with you some simple ideas for making bento box meals and snacks fun for school, at home and on the go.

So let's get started on our adventure in healthy eating...

Sherrie

P.S. Thanks to my book contributors Maia, Daniela, Sally, Nina and Cristi for making **Yum! Healthy Bento Lunches for Kids**, an awesome reference guide for busy parents of young children. I hope you will check out their blogs and websites for more healthy and creative school lunch ideas.

What is a Bento?

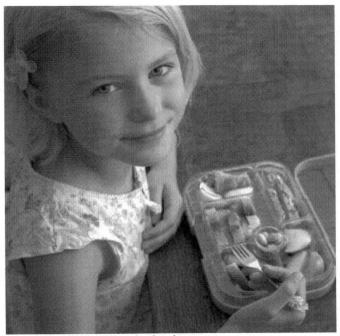

Photo courtesy of www.yumboxlunch.com

So just what is a bento? It is a type of meal efficiently packed in a box. Therefore, a healthy bento box *(that appeals to both kids and parents)* would be one that is both visually appealing and nutritionally balanced.

While the word itself is Japanese, this type of compact lunch container *(with its divided sections or compartments)* is similar in nature to the Indian *tuffin*, the Korean *dosirak*, or the Filipino *baon* lunch.

The term "bento" or "obento" refers to a packed meal in Japanese whereas the "bento-bako" refers to the lunch container itself.

Creative Menu Ideas

*Whole grain waffles cut into fingers and served alongside yogurt for dipping.

*Fresh bread sticks with pizza sauce for dipping.

*A sandwich on a stick. Alternate cubes of meat, cheese and bread on a short skewer *(cut off the sharp end).*

*Use large pieces of lettuce *(instead of a tortilla)* to wrap up sandwich fillings.

*Cut a bagel into cubes and pack with a flavored cream cheese for dipping *(add a little sour cream or mayonnaise to turn it into more of a dip).*

*Chop up a mixture of your child's favorite vegetables *(raw or cooked),* blend with a little salsa and pack in a pita along with some shredded lettuce and grated cheese.

*Be creative with sandwich filling combinations e.g. cream cheese and jam or egg salad and cucumbers.

*Pack a flat bottomed ice cream cone and have your kids fill it with tuna, salmon, egg or chicken salad.

*Make your own trail mix *(dried fruit and cereal)* and pack it alongside some yogurt and a banana.

Tip: *Getting kids to help in the kitchen makes food fun and by providing healthy ingredients and letting our kids help with the prep work, based on their age and skills; we encourage a love of healthy eating. When new foods are made together, chances are greater your kids will actually try the food they've helped to make.*

Why Use a Bento Box?

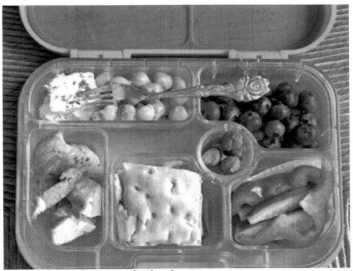

Photo courtesy of www.yumboxlunch.com

Inspired by the Greek cuisine, this simple lunch is accented by oregano and olive oil. It features a grilled chicken breast *(seasoned with olive oil and powdered oregano)*, red pepper and cucumber slices, feta cheese and chickpeas *(flavored with olive oil and dried oregano)* and flat bread. Rounding out the lunch are blueberries and toasted hazelnuts.

If you're looking to reduce your family's carbon footprint, a bento box container is a great way to go. It saves you money by eliminating the need for plastic lunch bags and wrap, multiple containers and store bought pre-packaged foods. Also think about how lunch box systems like the Yumbox make packing leftovers and other fresh foods more attractive.

The more appealing we can make our children's lunches, the greater the chance they will eat all of it.

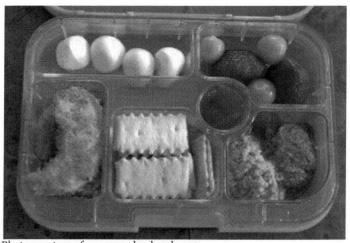

Photo courtesy of www.yumboxlunch.com

Homemade chicken strips take center stage in this school lunch. Serve this kid favorite alongside mozzarella cheese balls, crackers, homemade pesto *(basil and artichoke)*, physallis and strawberries *(or other favorites)* and you've got a lunch that offers up great appeal. Of course, you can't forget the ketchup for dipping.

Plus, since a lot of kids aren't into sandwiches, a bento box styled lunchbox presents a great opportunity to plan meals *(and leftovers)* your children really enjoy.

Personally, I've found serving up lunch in a bento box has encouraged me to do more baking and batch cooking on the weekend so my family has lots of choices for weekday lunches.

Buying in bulk and cooking up large batches of whole grain pasta, quinoa and rice in advance, along with preparing fresh fruits and vegetables while I'm making the dinner meal the night before, saves me a great deal of time. By baking more, I can help limit the amount of sugar my family consumes and I also save money by not buying as many packaged snacks and desserts.

What's in a Serving?

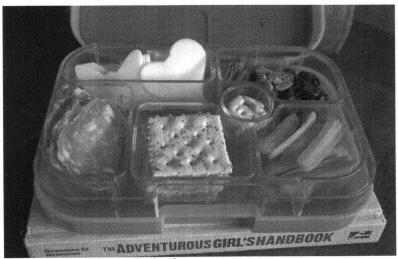

Photo courtesy of www.yumboxlunch.com

This lunch is a good example of typical serving sizes. It features 2 ounces each of mozzarella and salami, a handful of olive crackers and 1/2 cup of sliced baby carrots. For a treat, there's a small mixture of pecans and dried cranberries alongside a few sweet alphabet crackers.

It's always a challenge to know what to feed kids every day and registered dietitian, Sally Kuzemchak shares some insight into not only what we should be feeding our kids but also some good samples of serving sizes.

Aside from being a registered dietitian, Kuzemchak has a Master's degree in dietetics, is founder of a nutrition-based blog www.realmomnutrition.com *(Tales from the trenches. Advice for the real world)* and has years of experience writing about nutrition for magazines.

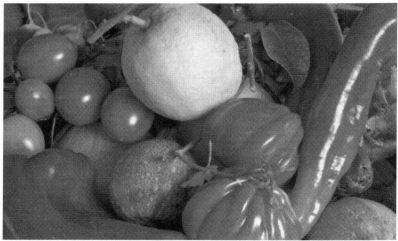

Photo courtesy of www.yumboxlunch.com

Fruits and Vegetables

We all want to get our kids to eat more fruits and vegetables but the challenge is often how, as well as how much, we should be serving up at each meal.

According to Kuzemchak, you should aim to feed toddlers 2 servings of fruits and vegetables per day, 2 to 3 for preschoolers, and 2 to 4 servings daily for school aged children.

Any fruit or 100% fruit juice counts as part of the 'Fruit' group, though whole food is preferred. Fruits may be fresh, canned, frozen, or dried, and may be whole, cut-up, or pureed.

The same goes for any vegetable or 100% vegetable juice, counting as a member of the 'Vegetable' group. Vegetables may be raw or cooked; fresh, frozen, canned, or dried/dehydrated; and may be whole, cut-up, or mashed.

"Try to divide the servings fairly equally between the two *(the fruits and vegetables categories)*. But if you have a

18

picky eater, set this minimum goal: offer at least one serving of dark-green or orange veggies daily. They have unique disease-preventing compounds," says Kuzemchak.

One of my favorite ways to get more vegetables into my children is to keep a see-thru container of cut-up vegetables handy in the refrigerator for both packing in school lunches and as quick grab and go snacks.

I also try to keep a good supply of seasonal fruits available in the refrigerator and in a fruit bowl on the kitchen counter so my family is always surrounded by a variety healthy eating options.

Ultimately, though I've found that making fresh garden and fruit salads is the best way to ensure that my family members get not only sufficient serving amounts but also a variety of fruits and vegetables in their diets. While salads are popular in our home, chances are greater they won't be prepared unless I either make them myself or have all the ingredients ready to go for quick assembly.

Fruit and vegetable serving examples:

Strawberries *(8 large)*

Seedless grapes *(32)*

Baby carrots *(12)*

Any fresh fruit or vegetable *(1 cup)*

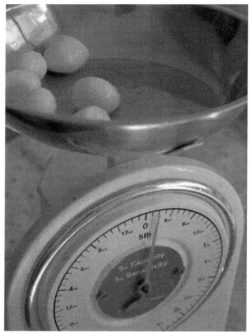

Photo courtesy of www.yumboxlunch.com

Use a food scale like this one to measure out serving sizes such as the 2 ounces of mozzarella balls pictured.

Dairy

One of my favorite ways to ensure my kids get their daily requirement of dairy is to pack a fruit or vegetable dip made of Greek yogurt in their school lunches.

According to Kuzemchak, your goal for dairy is 2 servings for toddlers, followed by 2 to 2 ½ servings for preschoolers, and 3 servings daily for school aged children.

All fluid milk products and many foods made from milk are considered part of the "Dairy' group. Foods made from milk that retain their calcium content are part of this food group. Likewise, foods made from milk that have little to no calcium, such as cream cheese, cream, and butter are not. That said calcium-fortified soy milk and other fortified non-dairy milks are part of the 'Dairy' group.

"If your kid is a milk lover, it'll be no problem for her to get the 800 milligrams of calcium she needs daily for strong bones and teeth *(or just 500mg, if she's between 1 and 3)*. Otherwise, focus on low-fat yogurt, cheese, and non-dairy sources of calcium like kale and spinach," says Kuzemchak.

She recommends making sure your brands of non-dairy milk contains vitamin D, which, among many other things, helps kids absorb calcium.

Good dairy servings include:

Shredded cheese *(1/3 cup)*

Yogurt *(1 cup, natural)*

String cheese *(1 piece)*

Milk *(1 cup)*

Fortified orange juice *(1 cup)*

Tip: *Easy ways to increase the amount of dairy in your child's diet include; adding grated cheese to sandwiches and salads, using milk instead of water when making muffins and plain yogurt instead of mayonnaise when preparing pasta salads for school lunches.*

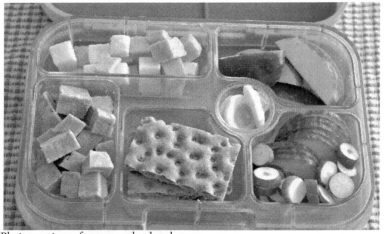

This protein packed lunch features 2 ounces of cheese, 3 ounces of ham, 2 Wasa crackers *(broken up)*, 1/2 cup sliced radishes and cucumber, 1 small apple *(sliced)* and a small treat.

Protein

With food allergies, nut-free classrooms as well as vegan and vegetarian dietary preferences, getting enough protein into your child can be a challenge but it doesn't have to be, if you implement some of the healthy bento box lunch ideas in this book.

All foods made from meat, poultry, seafood, beans and peas, eggs, processed soy products, as well as nuts and seeds are considered part of the 'Protein' group.

One of the best ways to incorporate protein in your child's school lunch is to use beans, peas or soy products as a main dish. Popular ideas include mixed bean salads, adding Garbanzo or kidney beans to a green salad, stir-fried tofu or recipes featuring flavorful combinations of rice and beans. And of course, you can't go wrong with hummus spread on pita wedges.

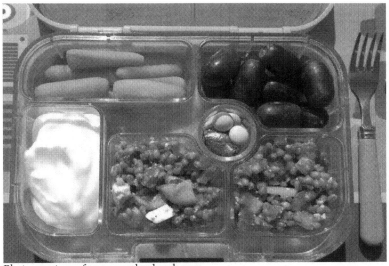

Photo courtesy of www.yumboxlunch.com

Looking for a nutrition-packed lunch for a child who typically has a hearty appetite? Consider packing a wheat berry salad like this one that features feta and fresh vegetables. Wheat berry is high in protein, carbs, fiber and even omega 3s. Rounding out this lunch are fresh grapes, baby carrots, mango yogurt and a small treat.

When it comes to protein, Kuzemchak recommends 2 servings of lean protein daily for toddlers, followed by 2 to 5 servings for preschoolers and 3 to 5 for school aged children.

"Protein-rich foods help build and repair every tissue in the body that kids need to grow. They also contain must-have nutrients -- like iron, zinc, and B vitamins," says Kuzemchak.

As for lean sources of protein, she suggests shopping for skinless chicken and turkey as well as cuts of meat with "loin" or "round" in its name. That way, you get protein minus the unhealthy fats.

Kuzemchak adds, "At least once a week, you should also serve fish and beans, which have nutrients that are not found in meat. Look for seafood such as shrimp, cod, and wild salmon that is low in mercury and is sustainably caught."

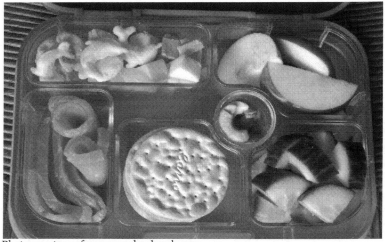

Photo courtesy of www.yumboxlunch.com

This packed lunch is a good example of how you can incorporate fish into your child's diet. Packed alongside strips of smoked salmon are Carr's crackers, a section of cheese cubes and fish crackers, chunks of cucumber, apple slices and a few cashews.

"I typically don't like to send fish in packed lunches, as my kids complain of the smell. But, smoked salmon, especially one that is very fresh and gently smoked, is a perfect lunch addition," says Maia Neumann, co-owner of Yumbox who packed the above lunch for her child.

Tip: *Among my favorite ideas for packing fish in school lunches is to combine fresh dill, chives and diced celery with canned salmon or tuna. Bind together with either natural yogurt or mayonnaise. Serve on a bed of lettuce or toss with cooked pasta shells or macaroni.*

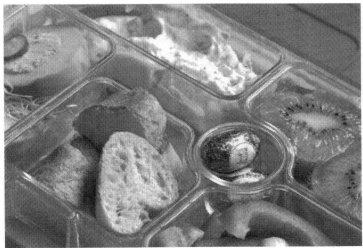

Photo courtesy of www.yumboxlunch.com

This Yumbox features 'pink' eggs *(details below)* topped with radish slices on a bed of sprouts alongside crusty bread, herbed cheese, pepper strips and more radishes with kiwi and chocolates for dessert.

"My kids are not huge egg eaters but they do like hard boiled eggs. Especially those left to soak in beet juice and acquire a pretty pink glow to them," says Neumann whose children regularly enjoy the benefits of a Yumbox packed meal.

Lean protein serving examples:

Egg *(1)*

Grilled chicken *(1/2 piece)*

Lean deli meat *(1 slice)*

Shrimp *(6)*

Tofu *(1/4 cup)*

25

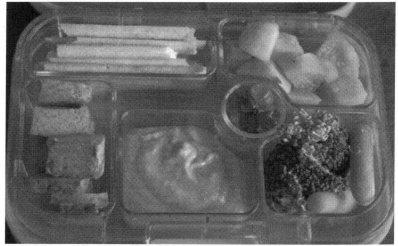

Photo courtesy of www.yumboxlunch.com

Vegetable proteins are a healthy option for school lunches. Pictured here is a good example of a protein-rich lunch that will help your child perform well and stay attentive during the school day. This lunch features tofu, peanut-ginger sauce, breadsticks, a medley of broccoli and carrots, melon cubes and a few gummy treats.

Healthy Fats

In addition to protein, children should have some healthy fats in their diets. Healthy fats can come in the form of salad dressings and oils like olive, canola, peanut or flax-seed as well as through nut and seed butters and via vegetables like avocados.

A nut-free butter or toasted soy spread like Safe 4 School WowButter is a good alternative for kids who love PB&J and are in nut-free classrooms.

Kuzemchak suggests you aim to serve toddlers 3 servings of healthy fats, preschoolers 3 to 4, and school aged kids 4 to 5.

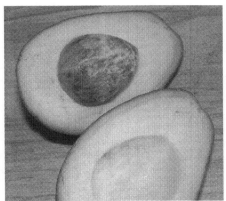

Photo courtesy of www.school-lunch-ideas.net

"All kinds of fats help kids grow, transport vitamins through the body, and provide vitamin E. But the unsaturated kind, like the type found in olive oil and avocado, protects kids' hearts by keeping their cholesterol level low. Though the research is still mixed, the saturated kind *(think butter)* may increase it. A government report recently found that 1 in 5 children has high cholesterol!" says Kuzemchak.

Good servings of healthy fats would be:

Peanut butter *(1 Tbsp.)*

Avocado *(1/2 medium)*

Sunflower seeds *(1/2 ounce)*

Nuts *(1/2 ounce e.g. 16 peanuts or 12 almonds)*

Olives *(4 large, sliced)*

Salad dressing *(2 Tbsp.)*

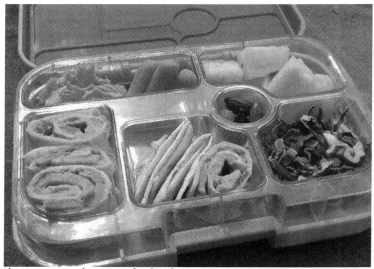

This balanced Yumbox features a good helping of grains in the way of baked ham pinwheels and extra tortilla strips for dipping in red pepper hummus. There are also carrots, shredded purple cabbage, fresh pineapple chunks, and almonds with chocolate as a treat.

Grains

School lunches are a great opportunity to serve up a good portion of your child's daily requirement of grains.

Grains run the gamut from bread and tortillas to pasta and cereal. Essentially any food made from wheat, rice, oats, cornmeal, barley or another cereal grain is classified as a grain product.

Kuzemchak recommends 3 grain servings a day for toddlers, 3 to 5 for preschoolers, and 5 for school aged children.

There are two categories of grains in the 'Grains' group – 'whole' and 'refined'.

"At least half of your kids' grain servings should be the unrefined type -- like whole wheat or oats -- because they contain more vitamin E, magnesium, and fiber than the processed kind. These 'whole' grains may also reduce your kids' risk of asthma, diabetes, and, later in life, heart disease," says Kuzemchak.

If your family is having trouble making the transition, she suggests buying breads and pastas made with a mix of whole and refined grains. Chances are good your kids won't even notice the change.

Serving examples of grains would be:

Whole wheat or corn tortilla *(small 6" size)*

Whole grain bread *(1 slice)*

Whole grain bagel *(1 mini)*

Brown rice *(1/2 cup, cooked)*

Whole grain pasta *(1/2 cup, cooked)*

Tip: *Some good ways to incorporate extra grains into your child's diet is to regularly send homemade cereal snack mixes, muffins and granola bars to school or pack whole grain cereal that can be mixed in with yogurt at lunchtime.*

The Dirty Dozen™
12 Most Contaminated

Apples
Celery
Cherries
Tomatoes
Cucumbers
Grapes
Hot Peppers
Nectarines *(Imported)*
Peaches
Potatoes
Spinach
Strawberries
Sweet Bell Peppers
*Plus, Collards and Kale as well as Summer Squash
and Zucchini*

The Clean Fifteen™
15 Least Contaminated

Asparagus
Avocado
Cabbage
Cantaloupe
Corn
Eggplant
Grapefruit
Kiwi
Mangos
Mushrooms
Onions
Papayas
Pineapple
Sweet Peas *(Frozen)*
Sweet Potatoes

Eating Organic

Whether or not to eat organic is a popular topic these days. Some families opt to eat only 100% organic produce, some prioritize their organic purchases and others simply eat the best they can based on their budget.

Personally, I believe the health benefits of a diet rich in fruits and vegetables outweigh the risks of pesticide exposure. That said, I always keep the EWG's (*Environmental Working Group*) Shopper's Guide to Pesticides™ guide top of mind when buying produce.

My aim is to reduce my family's exposure to pesticides as much as possible. While I don't avoid all conventionally grown produce, I do believe it is important to prioritize my purchases and to know which fruits and vegetables have the most pesticide residues and are the most important to buy organic.

Keeping a copy of The Shopper's Guide to Pesticides in Produce™ on hand when shopping will assist you in making wiser choices and can significantly lower your family's pesticide intake by helping you avoid or at the very least, limit the 12 most contaminated fruits and vegetables and select the least contaminated produce.

For your convenience, I've included a copy of the two EWG lists on page 30.

Visit http://www.ewg.org/foodnews/ to *download a PDF version of the guide* or an app for your smart phone.

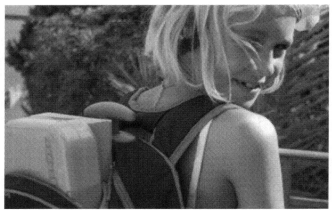

Did you know that one school-age child using a disposable lunch generates 67 pounds of waste per school year?

According to www.wastefreelunches.org, parents spend $4.02 per day by packing their child a "disposable" lunch, compared to on average $2.65 per day to pack a waste-free lunch.

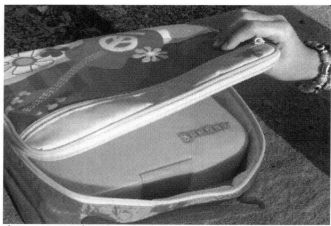

Picky Eater Solutions

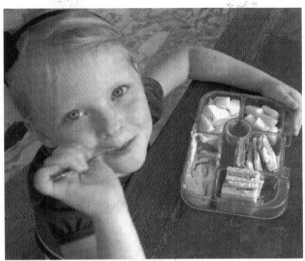

Photo courtesy of www.yumboxlunch.com

"Simple is better for picky eaters," says Neumann. "Don't overcomplicate their lunch. Just make sure it's the best quality you can find."

Even though children may be selective eaters, you still want to present them with lean meats and other sources of protein like beans *(black or kidney),* tofu, chickpeas, tempeh and quinoa as well as organic fruits and vegetables *(or ones with a skin that can be easily peeled).*

When shopping for dairy products opt for fresh milk, cheese, Greek yogurt and the like.

As for grains, focus more on brown versus white but be creative in how you present it.

The goal is to focus on quality versus quantity and to aim to get the best types of foods into your child.

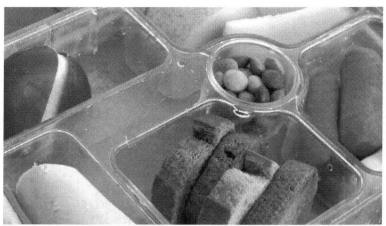

Photo courtesy of www.yumboxlunch.com

Pack a lunch featuring your children's favorite finger foods e.g. cheese, lean deli meat, cut-up fruits and vegetables, dense whole grain bread and a little treat like a few Smarties.

Children who are picky may be tempted by the attractive presentation of a variety of quality foods that don't touch as well as how the food is prepared. This is where a bento box container like Yumbox comes in real handy.

For many kids, bento boxes are all about fun. This type of lunch container lends itself to the enjoyment of a wider selection of foods because of the multiple sections.

Packing a bento box lunch for your child also doesn't have to be labor intensive. Adding cute food picks *(or other bento accessories)* in addition to a little container of dip for fresh fruits and veggies may be all you need to keep school lunches from coming home untouched.

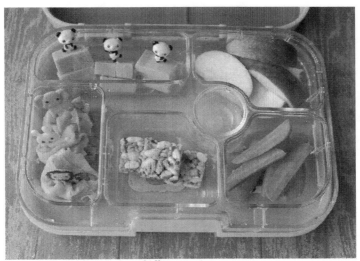

Photo courtesy of www.mamabelly.com

Food picks, like these adorable animal ones in this Yumbox lunch packed by Nina Holstead of www.Mamabelly.com , are a popular way to add an element of fun to school lunches and snacks. This kid-friendly snack/lunch features popular finger foods like nitrate free ham, cheese cubes, apples slices, carrot sticks and Naturebox cranberry almond bites.

When packing a bento box lunch, not only think balance, but also nutritional value. You also want to create a visual lunch that includes a variety of colors and textures.

By focusing on variety, lunches are more interesting. The chances are greater that interesting lunches will get eaten. And, the goal is always to provide our children with the energy and nutrients they need to grow, play, learn and stay healthy.

Bento boxes work towards achieving that goal by helping you pack a healthier, more balanced meal *(or snack)* for school classrooms as well as other times when your family is on the go.

35

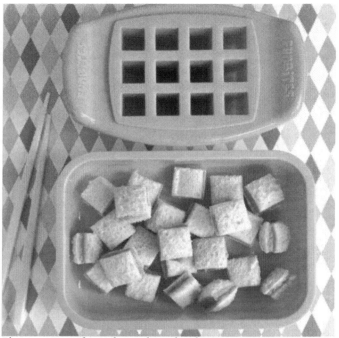

Photo courtesy of www.bentonbetterlunches.com

Offer up bite-sized meals

There's no doubt about it, little children love little things. Taking a couple of extra minutes to creatively cut up our children's foods into bite sized pieces can really make or break the appeal of school lunches.

Here's a fun school lunch idea from Cristi Messersmith of www.bentonbetter.lunches.com to combine chopsticks and mini sandwiches made with FunBites Squares sandwich cutters.

Messersmith, who has perfected the knack of using Fun-Bites to cube *(peanut butter or nut-free butter)* sandwiches for school lunches without making a mess, offers the following how-to suggestions.

Step 1:

Spread your selected butter on a slice of bread and then set it aside.

Step 2:

Take another slice of bread and partially press the Fun-Bites cutter into it, keeping the framework of the squares intact.

Step 3:

Lift the cutter with the bread pieces still stuck in the cutter and place it on top of the slice of bread coated with peanut or nut-free butter.

Step 4:

Press the FunBites cutter all the way through to the bottom slice and rock the cutter back and forth.

Step 5:

Use the popper *(that comes with the cutter)* to pop out the perfect mini sandwich cubes without the mess.

Voila! A lunch made for a kid and a pair of chopsticks!

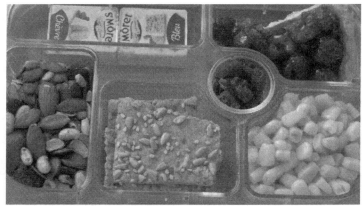

Photo courtesy of www.yumboxlunch.com

Does your child eat like a bird?

The fact is some children have small appetites and just like to nibble on food.

Consistent food exposure is one of the best ways to encourage a selective eater to eat healthier, and hopefully more, if they typically eat very little.

Research shows that children will voluntarily start eating a greater variety of food when they are exposed to multiple choices over a long period of time.

While I don't advocate force feeding a child who is healthy and growing well, I do recommend incorporating not only variety into school lunches and snacks but also adding in a few new items for your child to try on a consistent basis.

Tip: *Once you find something your children like, experiment with different variations e.g. if a classic turkey sandwich is a favorite, mix it up by making a turkey wrap with cream cheese and dried cranberries or turkey salad with celery and mayo.*

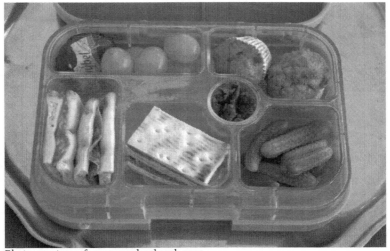

Photo courtesy of www.yumboxlunch.com

Quick and Easy

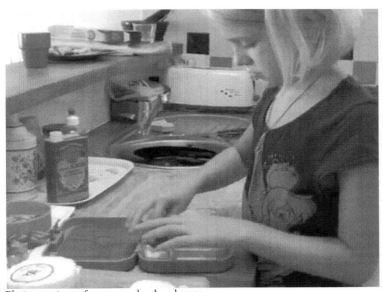

Photo courtesy of www.yumboxlunch.com

When you're pressed for time you can't beat quick and easy lunches and snacks. Bento boxes that can be assembled in less than 10 minutes are best for most families.

The key to quick and easy is to plan ahead, shop in advance so you have a good selection of fresh produce, meat, dairy etc. on hand. Where possible, do as much prep work as you can in advance.

Keeping lunch containers and accessories handy and organized will save you a lot of time. The trick is to be able to quickly find what you need when you need it.

Ideally, you want to keep everything you require for school lunches, close to the point of use. Keep tools like frequently used sandwich cutters, food picks etc. easily accessible in drawers and cupboards.

Messersmith whose creative bento box lunches can be found on her blog, www.bentonbetterlunches.com is a master of not only coming up with innovative school lunch ideas but she also has some accessory storage tips to share.

Her lunch prep and storage station is highly organized and efficient which lends itself well to her creativity and ease of making fun but also nutritious lunches for her three children.

By dedicating a corner of her kitchen to school related tools and supplies, Messersmith has created a work area where everything she needs for packing school lunches is close at hand.

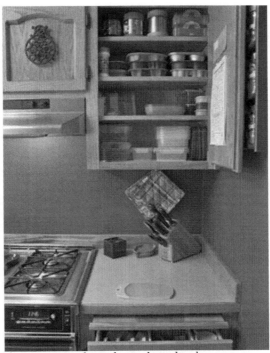
Photo courtesy of www.bentonbetterlunches.com

A Place for Everything

The kitchen cupboard pictured in the above photo holds Messersmith's containers and muffin tins. That said, a few items are missing from the photo as the picture was taken during a school day when certain supplies were in use.

The interior of the cupboard door is put to good use to keep hot lunch menus and lunch money account online access information handy.

The small green cutting board on the counter is typically stored on top of the tackle box of mini cutters and food picks in the drawer just below the pull-out cutting board.

41

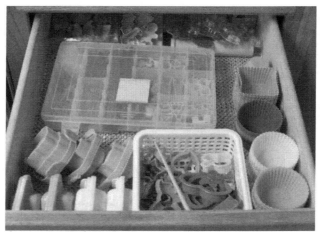

Photo courtesy of www.bentonbetterlunches.com

According to Messersmith, the above drawer also holds her muffin cups, egg molds, and various mini cutters and small tools. She also likes to keep Post-It notes in this drawer as well as she sometimes likes to stick a note on a container at night to remind herself the next morning what she wants to pack in it. As with most families, mornings can be pretty chaotic in the Messersmith household.

"I don't have time to stare at an empty container wracking my brain about what to put in it," she adds.

When creating fun sandwiches for her kids, Messersmith uses a variety of cutters including Lunch Punches *(her favorite)* and other cookie cutters like those made by Wilton.

To store all her favorite Lunch Punch sandwich cutters, Messersmith has creatively repurposed a tiered drawer spice rack and keeps everything handy in her school lunch preparation area. Now, all it takes is a quick glance for her to locate the cutter she needs.

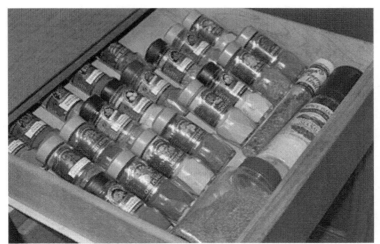

Above is a 'before' photo of Messersmith's spice drawer and below is an 'after' photo of her Lunch Punch storage centre. Each of the five tiers is the perfect width and depth to hold four sandwich cutters, and they can be stacked two deep.

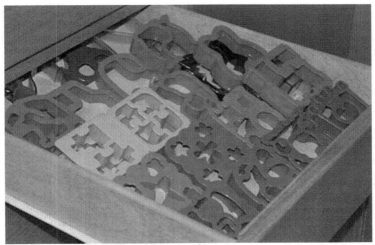

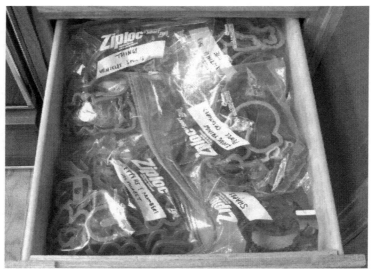
Photo courtesy of www.bentonbetterlunches.com

To keep a handle on all her cookie cutters, Messersmith sorted them into categories and put them into individual plastic bags, which she in turn, labelled with a description of what was inside.

One of the best ways she's found to keep frequently used cookie cutters front and centre is to rotate the bags so the shapes most appropriate to the season, are on top.

Messersmith adds, it also helps that the Wilton cutters she has are color coded e.g. the Halloween cutters are all orange, the number cutters are blue, the spring and East-er shapes are yellow etc. which makes it really easy for her to find the one she needs quickly.

To learn more about the specific tools Messersmith uses, (and to find out where she now stores her spices) drop by her blog www.bentonbetterlunches.com

Lunches

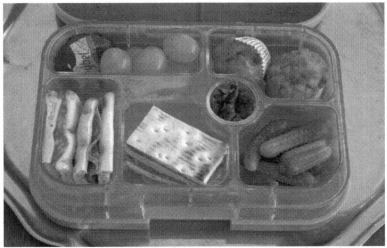

Photo courtesy of www.yumboxlunch.com

Flatbread Salami Lunch

Flat breads with salami, cornichon pickles *(gherkins)*, apple walnut muffins, grapes, Babybel cheese and dried cranberries make up this Yumbox lunch.

Tip: *Looking to pack apple slices in your child's lunch but don't want them to turn brown by lunchtime? Try soaking them in orange juice, ginger ale or club soda for a few minutes first, before patting dry and packing in your child's lunch.*

Also, if you find you have several apples that have started to wilt, consider making up a batch of apple sauce, quick bread or muffins and freezing them for a healthy addition to your children's lunch boxes.

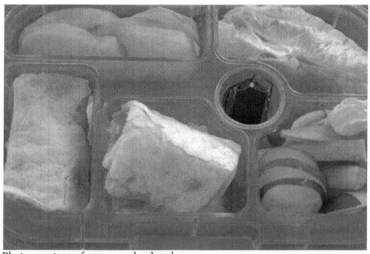

Photo courtesy of www.yumboxlunch.com

Mortadella Wrap Lunch

Mortadella takes top billing in this child's lunch. Here, the mortadella wrap is cut into three parts and is served alongside smoked mozzarella and a finger salad of lettuce, radishes and carrots. For a sweet finish, orange sections and dark chocolate with almonds has been added.

Sandwich wraps have greater appeal to most kids than ordinary bread sandwiches and cutting the wraps into smaller pieces typically make them more enjoyable.

Tip: *Keep things interesting by varying the types and flavors of the wraps you use e.g. soft corn tortillas or whole grain pitas sliced in half and rolled up. Also look for a variety of flavored soft tortillas e.g. tomato basil or spinach. In addition to switching up the taste of the wraps, different flavors also add a nice variety of color to school lunches.*

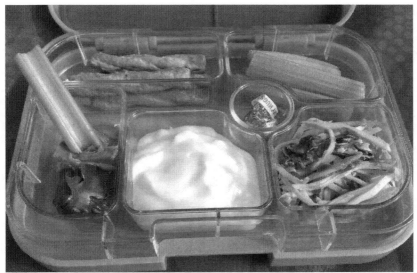

Photo courtesy of www.yumboxlunch.com

A 'Full of Crunch' Lunch

Kids often like the appeal of a crunchy lunch. This lunch features shredded veggies, celery sticks, pretzel twists with Nutella and peanut butter for dipping alongside banana yogurt.

"The tooth fairy comes and suddenly some healthy favorites are no longer chewable! My daughter loves salads, but since more than a few of those little teeth have gone missing, flat leaves are hard to chew. She prefers crunchy. So a staple the past few weeks has been shredded veggies *(carrots, broccoli, cauliflower, purple cabbage),*" says Neumann, who adds that she buys these vegetables already shredded for the convenience.

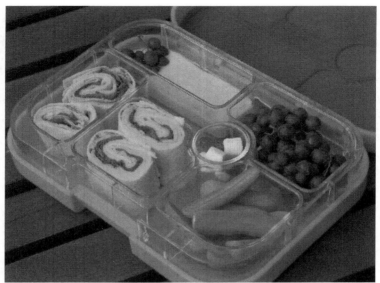

Photo courtesy of www.yumboxlunch.com

Pinwheel Lunch

One of the best ways to pack sandwich wraps in your children's lunches is to cut them into pieces so they resemble pinwheels.

Sandwich wraps are also a great way to incorporate extra vegetables into a child's diet.

"I tend to use shredded purple cabbage for crunch, avocado to add a creamy consistency and arugula for a little green spice," says Neumann. "Those veggies go with pretty much anything."

Tip: *Spread cream cheese on a soft tortilla and then toss on a handful of raisins or other dried fruits like cherries or blueberries. Enjoy alone or pair with lean turkey or chicken.*

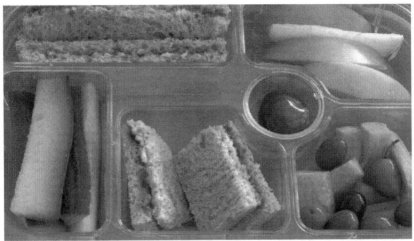
Photo courtesy of www.yumboxlunch.com

Toasted Lunch

I'm sure all parents can relate to finding enjoyment in the packing of healthy and creative kids' lunches at the beginning of the school year but as time goes by, we get busy and our enthusiasm for packing lunches often disappears as we run out of fresh new ideas and ways to vary the ingredients.

School lunches don't have to be fancy. Simple meals like toast and jam served alongside fresh fruit and veggies are quite acceptable.

In this case, toasted whole wheat bread, spread with butter and plum preserves is paired with cucumber spears, cut-up carrots, olives, apple slices and two chocolate hearts for a treat.

A lunch like this is familiar and should appeal to young taste buds.

49

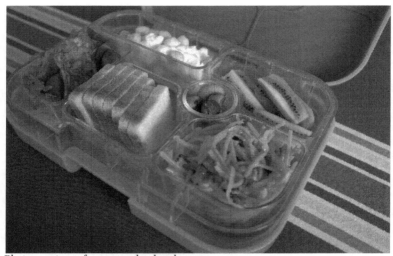

Photo courtesy of www.yumboxlunch.com

Carrot Salad Lunch

Salami slices and little toasts take top billing in this Yumbox lunch that also features yogurt with cereal puffs, carrot salad, cashew nuts and sliced kiwi.

To make the carrot salad, shred two carrots and then add some raisins, honey, olive oil, lemon, and mint to taste.

Tip: *If your children love carrots, consider the many different ways of preparing them. You can slice carrots into coins, cut them into half-moons, into sticks, or turn them into fun shapes using heavy-duty vegetable cutters. Cut thick baby carrots lengthwise for variety.*

Other ideas for creatively packing carrots in your kids' lunches include; mixing grated carrots with cabbage and apples for a coleslaw, tossing some (along with a handful of raisins) in a favorite dressing as a pita filling, or combine with cream cheese and stuff into celery.

How to Make Carrot Hearts

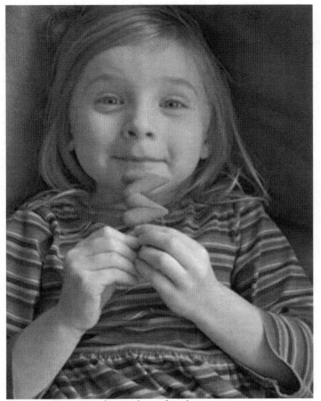

Photo courtesy www.bentonbetterlunches.com

To make these adorable carrot hearts you first start with baby carrots which are ideal because they already have rounded ends. Select the most 'plump' ones in the package as they are less likely to split when you skewer them.

Thanks to the creativity of Cristi Messersmith from www.bentonbetterlunch.com for the idea and related photos.

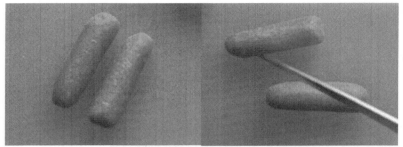

Slice the carrots on the diagonal. Then flip over one of the pieces of diagonally sliced carrot.

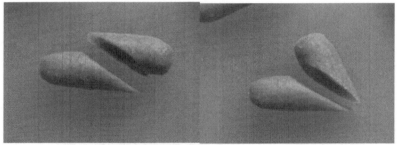

The two halves make a heart. Skewer the pieces of carrot so that the flat ends fit flush.

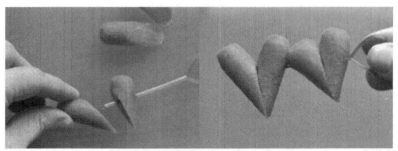

Viola! Two carrot hearts ideal for packing in your child's bento box lunch.

Carrot Hearts for Toddlers

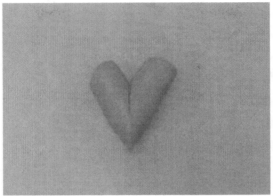

Photo courtesy www.bentonbetterlunches.com

For younger children, here's a step-by-step for making carrot hearts without using picks.

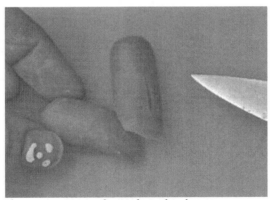

Photo courtesy www.bentonbetterlunches.com

Follow the previous steps for cutting the baby carrots on the diagonal and flipping them over. Next, you want to cut slits in the carrot heart halves (*where the picks would go through if you were using picks*).

53

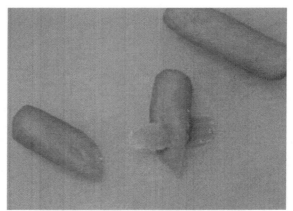
Photo courtesy www.bentonbetterlunches.com

Then cut a sliver from another carrot and then use it in lieu of a pick. Push the sliver into the slits to connect the two pieces. Now simply trim any pieces left sticking out.

Snacks

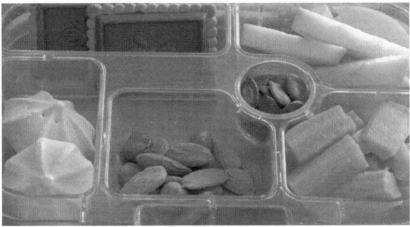

Photo courtesy of www.yumboxlunch.com

After School Snacks

Whether at home or on the go after class, after school snacks help keep hunger at bay until dinner time.

Fruit, nuts, seeds, cut up vegetables and occasionally sweet snacks like dark chocolate cookies and meringues make great snacks for hungry kids.

When packing snacks for after school enjoyment, don't forget to include a bottle of water to keep your children hydrated. This is particularly important if your kids are participating in after school sports.

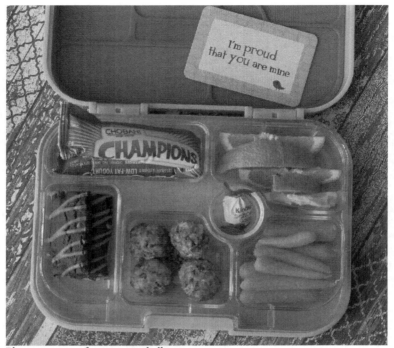

Photo courtesy of www.mamabelly.com

Energy Snacks

This energy packed Yumbox features a Chobani Champions blueberry tube alongside oranges, carrots, no bake energy bites, a protein cereal bar and a small treat.

Tip: *Add an element of fun to your kids' bento boxes by including a silly joke or riddle to share, colorful stickers with cheery messages or sayings, or tuck in a novelty pencil or eraser.*

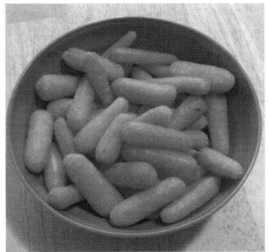

Photo courtesy of www.school-lunch-ideas.net

Healthy Snack Ideas

Healthy snacking occasionally is one thing but snacks should never replace a meal. One of the best ways to ensure that our children are healthy snackers is to provide them with portion sized snack options.

For instance, you may want to store snack-sized containers of homemade snack mixes in your pantry.

Make your own snack mixes from dry whole grain cereal, popcorn *(for older children),* dried fruit as well as unsalted nuts or seeds.

Alternatively, supply a bunch of different ingredients and let your kids create their own snack packs.

Another good snack idea for kids on the go is to offer up a single-serving container of yogurt alongside individually wrapped string cheese.

Following is a collection of some of my favorite snack combo ideas:

*Hummus and whole grain crackers

*Baby carrots and broccoli with low-fat ranch dip.

*Tortilla chips with tomato salsa and black beans

*Oil-popped popcorn sprinkled with grated Parmesan cheese.

*Lean deli meat wrapped around an apple wedge.

*Quick veggie pizza made by topping half a whole wheat English muffin with spaghetti sauce, chopped vegetables and grated mozzarella cheese. Melt in a microwave or toaster oven.

*Fruit kabobs featuring chunks of melons, oranges, grapes, strawberries etc. on skewers.

*Veggie kabobs made with zucchini, cucumber, squash, sweet peppers, tomatoes and the like on skewers and served alongside a favorite dip.

*Frozen fruit pops made by inserting sticks into chunks of banana, melon, strawberries etc. before freezing.

Tip: *Here's a 'fun with food' idea. Offer up some healthy snack ingredients and encourage your kids to create some food art e.g. supply them with carrot sticks or celery as well as thin slices of apple, a small container of peanut butter (or a nut-free butter) along with some dried fruit and grapes cut in half and get them to create a butterfly. For more 'fun with food' ideas visit www.pinterest.com/schoollunches*

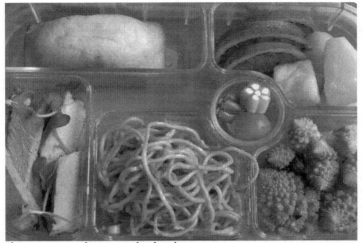

Photo courtesy of www.yumboxlunch.com

Using Leftovers

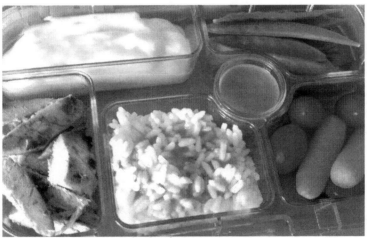

Photo courtesy of www.yumboxlunch.com

Besides a bento box, what makes packing lunches extra easy? If you answered 'leftovers' then you'll probably enjoy this section of the book featuring favorite ideas from the night before.

Whether you pack a repeat of last night's dinner or use the leftover ingredients to make an entirely new meal, having some leftovers on hand is an excellent place to start.

Menu planning as well as batch cooking are two great ways to ensure that you have leftovers ready for packing in weekday lunches.

Topping my list of favorite leftover ingredients is cooked pasta, quinoa and rice that can be reincarnated into a variety of flavorful salads. Sources of protein like hard boiled eggs from breakfast or roast ham or grilled chicken from dinner the night before, are other good lunch box foods you may want to plan ahead for.

And don't forget the veggies. Not all vegetables you pack need to be raw. If you have steamed broccoli, beans, carrots and the like from dinner the night before, by all means pack them.

Another popular way to use leftovers is to package them up in advance e.g. save some rice from dinner on Saturday for lunch on Monday. Likewise, turn leftover turkey from Sunday dinner into turkey salad on Tuesday. Leftovers don't have to be used the following day *(just within a few days)*. The trick is to label and package leftovers you have a plan for, otherwise when you go to use them, they could be gone.

Following is a collection of bento box ideas that creatively use leftovers for lunches...

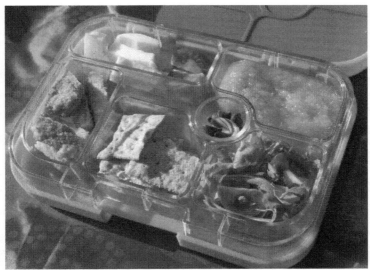

Photo courtesy of www.yumboxlunch.com

Leftover Lunch #1

Some foods taste even better the next day. Because of this it makes sense to plan to have leftovers. A leftover lunch is also one that can quickly be assembled.

"There are some foods I prefer more the next day. Chicken and pork cutlets are two of those foods. They taste great cold or at room temperature for a packed lunch," says Neumann. "I just have to be sure to make enough to have leftovers!"

This leftover lunch features bite-sized pieces of pork cutlet, applesauce, wheat herb crackers, Fontina cheese, as well as arugula and tomato salad. Today's treat is peppermint candy and chocolate morsels.

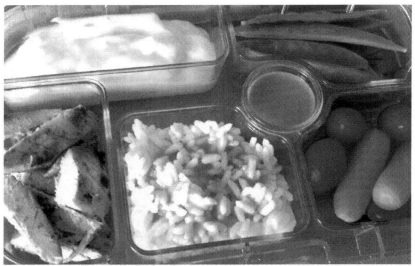

Photo courtesy of www.yumboxlunch.com

Leftover Lunch #2

As the kids grow and their appetites increase you may find fewer leftovers in which to make use of in the next day's lunch. The key is not only to plan for leftovers but take a minute to pack up a portion in your child's bento box right at dinner time and store in the refrigerator overnight. Packing lunch at dinnertime is not only efficient but it also saves you considerable time over the course of the week.

This quick and easy leftover lunch #2 features grilled chicken alongside rice and tomatoes, carrots and snow peas. Extra dipping sauce is included for drizzling on the rice and for dipping the vegetables in. The dessert is orange yogurt.

Tip: *If you children are still hungry at dinner time load them up with extra salad and/or steamed veggies.*

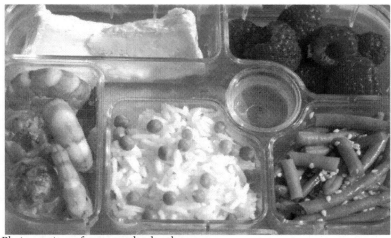

Photo courtesy of www.yumboxlunch.com

Asian Inspired Lunch #1

This Asian inspired lunch features a mini eggroll, steamed shrimp, rice with peas, steamed green beans with sesame seeds, camembert, raspberries and dipping sauce.

Tip: *You can make rice more appealing by adding some of your child's favorite vegetables to it.*

The same goes for the vegetables. Serve them up a little differently in your child's lunch box. Toss cooked beans in a favorite dressing e.g. balsamic vinaigrette or ranch dressing with some cooked and crumbled bacon mixed in. Alternatively, serve with toasted slivered almonds or roasted sesame seeds (as pictured).

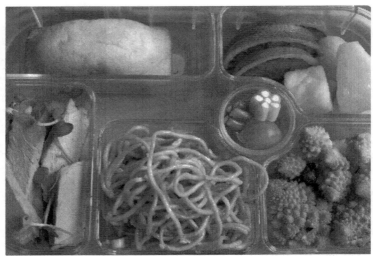
Photo courtesy of www.yumboxlunch.com

Asian Inspired Lunch #2

This second Asian inspired lunch features Asian noodles with scallions, ginger, and sesame oil alongside roasted pork with ginger and garlic, roasted romanesco, pineapple, blood orange slices, and yogurt-vanilla cake.

Celebrate different holidays by creating themed lunches. Here, Asian noodles celebrate the Year of the Snake. Fresh ginger was used with the noodles, pork and romanesco *(a type of broccoli)* to create a unifying taste.

Ginger has a lot of beneficial health properties.

Tip: *The life of fresh ginger can be extended by freezing it in a plastic bag between uses.*

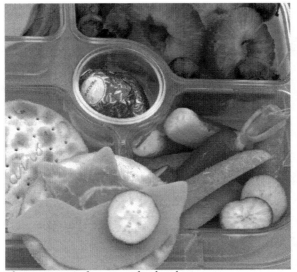

Fun with Shapes

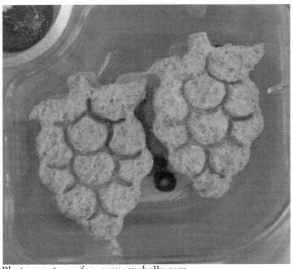

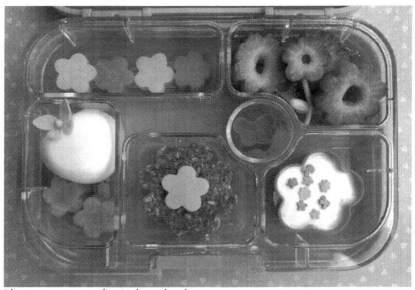

Photo courtesy www.bentonbetterlunches.com

Berry-licious Garden Lunch

This fresh and colorful lunch from Cristi Messersmith of www.bentonbetterlunches.com features a hard-cooked egg with a butterfly pick, blossom-shaped carrots, cheddar cheese, oatmeal bar, and strawberries. Blossom-sprinkled yogurt is also packed in a flower shaped container. The treat of the day is two gummy butterflies.

Tip: *Looking for a different way to present eggs in your children's lunches? Consider using egg molds like those made by Kotobuki that come in a variety of kid-friendly shapes like bunnies, bears, fish, cars, stars, and hearts.*

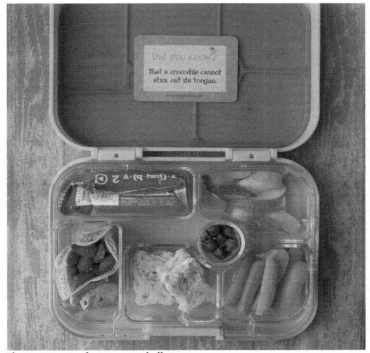

Photo courtesy of www.mamabelly.com

A Beary Delicious Lunch

This healthy Yumbox lunch packed by Nina Holstead of www.mamabelly.com for her son who is in first grade, features a Chobani Champions tube, apple bunnies, Naturebox cinnamon almonds, two mini chocolate chip cookies, two bear peanut butter and honey sandwiches, carrots and a few chocolate chips.

Tip: *Pack a water bottle in your child's lunch every day. A clean, reusable water bottle filled with fresh, filtered water will help your kids quench their thirst throughout the day and it saves them from having to drink from a shared water fountain.*

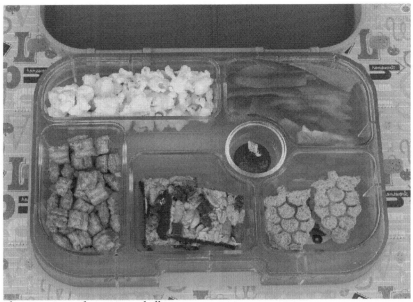

Photo courtesy of www.mamabelly.com

A Snack for Lunch

This child selected lunch from blogger Nina Holstead features popular menu items like two mini grape jelly sandwiches, sliced sweet peppers, Berry Blossoms cereal from Kashi, a cereal bar, popcorn and a Hershey kiss as a treat.

Tip: *When selecting beverages for school lunches, make it a habit to read the nutrition label. The Nutrition Facts label contains information about total sugars, fats, and calories and will help you make better choices*

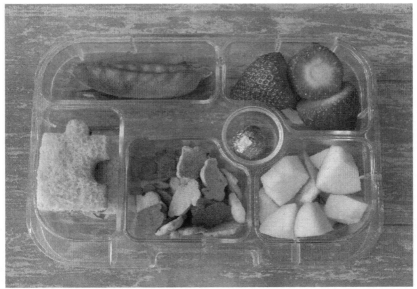

Photo courtesy of www.mamabelly.com

Puzzle Lunch

Puzzled about what to pack in your child's lunch? A variety of healthy foods cut up into chunks or made into different shapes using a variety of food cutters like those made for vegetables, cookies and sandwiches is usually a winner.

This Yumbox, packed for a 4 year old, is one of the many school lunch ideas featured on the www.mamabelly.com blog. It includes two puzzle piece sandwiches, steamed snow peas, strawberries, apples, some Annie's bunny cookies and a Hershey kiss to round out the meal.

Tip: *It's okay to switch up your child's beverages occasionally. Instead offering soda and other sugar laden beverages, add seltzer water to 1/2 cup of 100% fruit juice.*

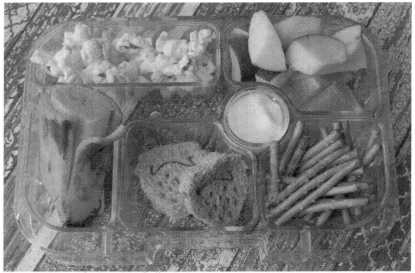

Photo courtesy of www.mamabelly.com

At Home Lunch

This www.mamabelly.com packed lunch for a 3 year old, features two mini strawberry jelly sandwiches (shaped like strawberries made with a cookie cutter stamp), half a banana, popcorn, apples, oranges, a small amount of vanilla yogurt to dip the apples in and a handful of pretzels.

Tip: *Clean sweep refrigerated foods once a week to make sure that the foods you are packing in your child's bento box are safe for consumption.*

Did you know? *If you don't rinse fresh vegetables and fruits under running water just before eating, cutting, or cooking; you risk transferring microbes from the outside to the inside. It is wise to rinse produce even if you just plan on peeling it before eating.*

Source: www.choosemyplate.gov

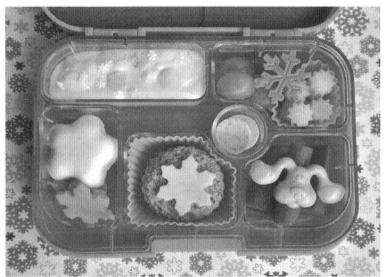

Photo courtesy www.bentonbetterlunches.com

Themed Lunches

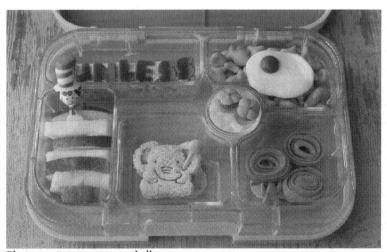

Photo courtesy www.mamabelly.com

There's no doubt about it, themed lunches are popular with kids, especially preschoolers and primary grade students.

Creating a themed lunch for your children is more about being creative and adding in fun elements than it is about spending hours making a masterpiece of food art.

Thanks to the popularity of bento boxes and related accessory items it is relatively easy to create a fun themed lunch with the supplies you have on hand.

Included in this 'Themed Lunches' section of the book are just a few ideas from bloggers Cristi Messersmith of www.bentonbetterlunches.com and Nina Holstead of www.mamabelly.com Be sure to check out both of their blogs for more of their creative ideas for school lunches.

Speaking of creative ideas for kids' lunches, Pinterest is a handy resource for fresh new ideas.

Check out our group 'School Lunch Ideas' board @ www.pinterest.com/schoollunches/school-lunch-ideas

(Email me @ Sherrie@school-lunch-idea.net and I'll invite you to share some of your own creative ideas.)

Additionally two of the best places to shop for decorative bento box accessories like food picks, cupcake rings, food cutters etc. are www.allthingsforsale.com (BentoUSA) and www.amazon.com

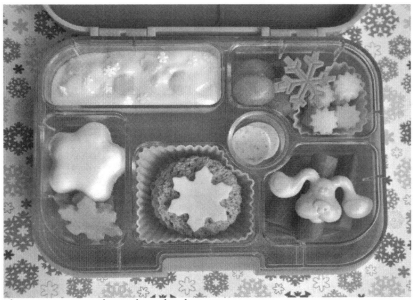
Photo courtesy www.bentonbetterlunches.com

Winter Blues Clues Lunch

This kid-friendly lunch by Messersmith is filled with fun and healthy foods like cheddar cheese snowflakes, a hard cooked egg blossom *(made with a star egg mold)* and a little white cheddar cheese sandwich on honey wheat bread. There's also yogurt with snowflake and blossom sprinkles as well as green grapes and Galia melon cut like bite-sized snowflakes *(with a snowflake cupcake pick for decoration)*. The carrot sticks are accented with a Blues Clues cupcake ring. The treat of the day is a couple of candy melts.

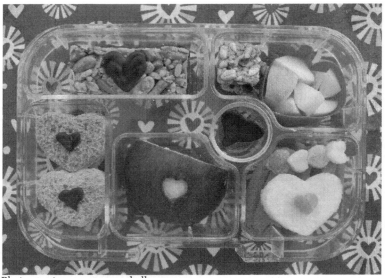

Photo courtesy www.mamabelly.com

I Love You Lunch

Whether it's Valentine's Day or any other day of the year, you want to send a little extra love in your child's lunch box, this creative meal may offer up some inspiration. For her youngest son, Holstead packed a cereal bar, mini heart sandwiches, a few Naturebox Cranberry Almond Bites, apple pieces, carrots with an apple and carrot heart, a mini apple skewer and half a red pear with a heart cut out. She also added a few chocolate hearts as well for decoration.

Tip: *Keep lunches interesting by packing the occasional theme lunch e.g. a color-coded lunch where you serve up only red or green foods.*

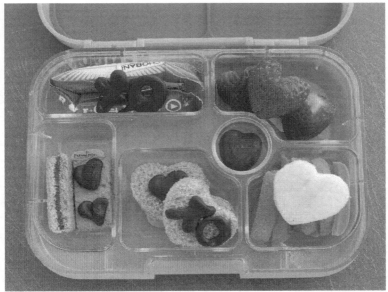

Photo courtesy www.mamabelly.com

Hugs and Kisses Lunch

Nothing says 'I love you' more than a packed lunch featuring heart-shaped food and a few hugs and kisses *(in this case, in the form of chocolate decorations).*

This Yumbox packed lunch by Holstead also includes a Chobani Champions strawberry tube, strawberry hearts, carrots with a big apple heart, mini sandwiches and a cereal yogurt bar.

Tip: *When making homemade treats, reduce the amount of sugar the recipe calls for and add dried fruit like apricots or raisins instead. Also substitute unsweetened applesauce or prune puree for half the amount of fat (e.g. butter or shortening) called for in the recipe.*

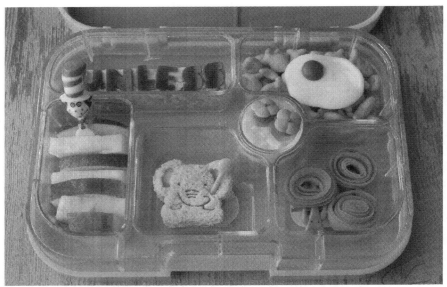

Photo courtesy www.mamabelly.com

Dr. Seuss Lunch

This Dr. Seuss themed lunch features creative details from The Cat in the Hat; One Fish, Two Fish; The Lorax and Horton Hears a Who since, lunch creator Holstead's daughter couldn't decide which her favorite book was.

Included is a cereal bar topped with fruit leather spelling out 'unless' from The Lorax, and goldfish crackers representing One Fish, Two Fish topped with green eggs. There is also Thing 1 and Thing 2 taking a bath in vanilla pudding, a Horton holding carrot tartuffolo trees *(carrot spirals)*, a speck sandwich and a small Cat in the Hat character tucked in with the apple slices.

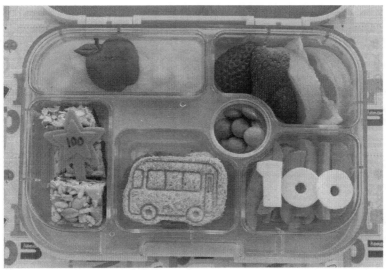
Photo courtesy www.mamabelly.com

100th Day of School Lunch

What a fun way to celebrate the 100th Day of School! This colorful themed lunch packed by Holstead made her first grader's day.

This lunch features a pepperoni 'bus' sandwich, a cereal bar, applesauce, strawberries and oranges, carrots with a cheese '100' and a few chocolate candies.

Did you know? *Children get the same calcium and other nutrients, but with fewer calories and less saturated fat by drinking low-fat (1%) or fat-free milk. For children who can't drink milk due to allergies or lactose intolerance, offer milk substitutes like calcium-fortified soy beverages instead.*

Source: www.choosemyplate.gov

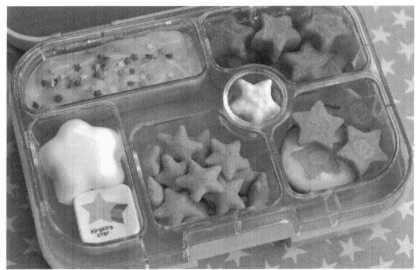

Photo courtesy www.bentonbetterlunches.com

Starry Lunch

What a fun lunch for preschoolers!

This 'starry' lunch packed by Messersmith features a molded star egg, yogurt with sprinkles, watermelon, carrots and cucumbers, whole grain crackers to dip in peanut butter *(in the star box)* and a couple of TJ's yogurt cookie stars for a treat.

Tip: *Encourage your child to eat lean proteins by packing low-sodium deli meats in school lunches, storing a selection of unsalted nuts in your pantry and by keeping hard-boiled eggs in the refrigerator ready for quick and easy snacking.*

Further Resources

Kids Food Adventure App

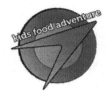

FREE app for iPhone/iPad

www.kidsfoodadventure.com/#

Choose My Food App

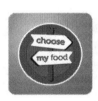

Customize your picky eater's journey to a healthy diet

www.kidsfoodadventure.com/choose-my-food#

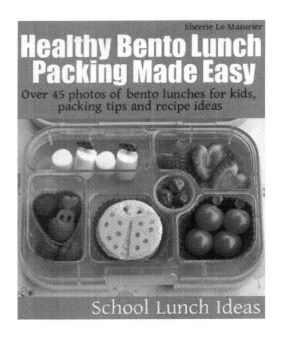

Healthy Bento Lunch Packing Made Easy

'Healthy Bento Lunch Packing Made Easy', is the second book in the School Lunch Ideas series and takes off where 'Yum! Healthy Bento Box Lunches for Kids' left off.

Also focusing on healthy eating for kids preschool to age 10, this book shares over 45 photos of bento box lunches, packing tips and recipe ideas.

This book is available via Amazon in both digital and paperback.

School Lunch Ideas

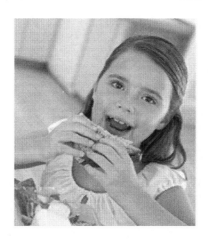

www.school-lunch-ideas.net

www.facebook.com/SchoolLunchIdeas

www.pinterest.com/schoollunches

Subsequent books in the 'School Lunch Ideas' series will explore different kinds of school lunch ideas, foods and themes.

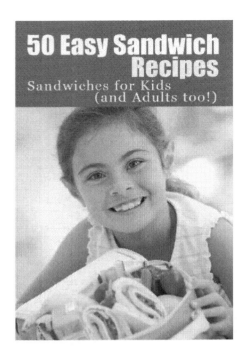

50 Easy Sandwich Recipes
Sandwiches for Kids
(and Adults Too!)

This quick and easy digest guide of sandwich recipe ideas by Sherrie Le Masurier features breads, buns, tortillas, pitas etc.

Discover ingredient combinations as well as creative ways to make sandwiches interesting for kids e.g. sandwich spirals and fingers.

This book is available via Amazon in both digital and paperback.

Contributors

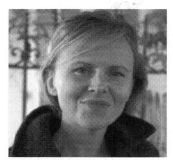

Maia Neumann

Maia Neumann is based in Southern France. She loves to cook, explore regional markets and is obsessively trying to get her kids to like tomatoes.

www.yumboxlunch.com

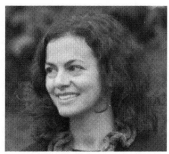

Daniela Devitt

After many years in Italy and New York City, Daniela Devitt now lives in Bucks County, PA. She is a master of thin crust pizza and loves sharing the kitchen with her kids.

www.yumboxlunch.com

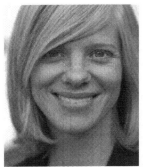

Sally Kuzemchak, MS, RD

Sally Kuzemchak, MS, RD, mom of two young kids, who tries to get everyone fed without losing her sanity or her sense of humor.

www.realmomnutrition.com

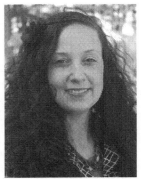

Nina Holstead

Nina Holstead is a military wife and a mom of four trying to make healthy and fun lunches while surviving the daily chaos. She's a coffee lover, bento enthusiast and always looking to learn more.

www.mamabelly.com

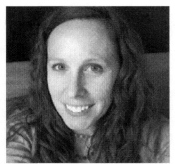

Cristi Messersmith

Cristi Messersmith is a busy military wife, and mom to five picky sproutlets, one with autism. In her spare time she enjoys... oh, who are we kidding, she doesn't have any spare time! Her blog chronicles her efforts to provide her family with nutritious, affordable, fun trash-free lunches for school and work.

www.bentonbetterlunches.com

About the Author

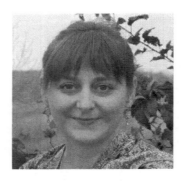

Sherrie Le Masurier is a busy mom and lifestyle writer who believes in serving up nutritional meals to her family. After learning about her daughter's intolerance to gluten and having experienced some food related health issues herself, Sherrie started www.school-lunch-ideas.net and www.how-to-live-gluten-free.com as a way to share healthy and creative food ideas.

Sherrie is also a professional organizer who helps parents better organize their home and family life via www.sherrielemasurier.com where she offers up smart solutions for busy families.

**For a complete list of books
By Sherrie Le Masurier visit
Sherrie's Author Page on Amazon**

Made in the USA
Charleston, SC
25 August 2015